The Plant-Based Diet Meal Plan

How-To Guide To Meal Plan To Eat Well Every Day, Lose Weight Fast And Get A Healthy Life With Simple, Healthy, Whole-Food Recipes To Kick-Start Healthy Eating

Jason Canon

TABLE OF CONTENTS

Introduction

Thank you very much for purchasing this book.

There are a lot of words going around about which diet is best for you. Despite this, many health and wellness communities will agree that those diets that emphasize fresh, whole ingredients, making sure to minimize the foods that are processed are the ones that are best for your overall well-being.

In this recipe book you will find dishes to prepare with fresh and healthy foods that, in addition to having a better taste, will help you on your weight loss journey.

Breakfast Recipes

Coconut Blackberry Breakfast Bowl

Preparation time: 15 minutes

Cooking time: 2 minutes

Servings: 2

Ingredients:

2 tbsp chia seeds

¼ cup coconut flakes

1 cup spinach

¼ cup of water

3 tbsp ground flaxseed

1 cup unsweetened coconut milk

1 cup blackberries

Directions:

Add blackberries, flaxseed, spinach, and coconut milk into the blender and blend until smooth. Fry coconut flakes in the pan for 1-2 minutes.

Pour berry mixture into the serving bowls and sprinkle coconut flakes and chia seeds on top. Serve immediately and enjoy.

Nutrition:

Calories 182

Fat 11.4 g

Carbohydrates 14.5 g

Protein 5.3 g

Cinnamon Coconut Pancake

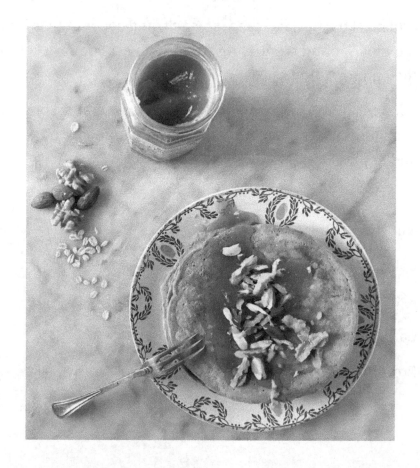

Preparation time: 15 minutes

Cooking time: 10 minutes

Servings: 1

Ingredients:

1/2 cup almond milk

1/4 cup coconut flour

2 tbsp egg replacer

8 tbsp water

1 packet stevia

1/8 tsp cinnamon

1/2 tsp baking powder

1 tsp vanilla extract

1/8 tsp salt

Directions:

Mix egg replacer and 8 tablespoons of water in a small bowl. Add all ingredients into the mixing bowl and stir until combined.

Spray pan with cooking spray and heat over medium heat. Pour the desired amount of batter onto the hot pan and cook until lightly golden brown. Flip pancake and cook within a few minutes more. Serve and enjoy.

Nutrition:Calories 110,Fat 4.3 g,Carbohydrates 10.9 g,

Protein 7 g

Flax Almond Muffins

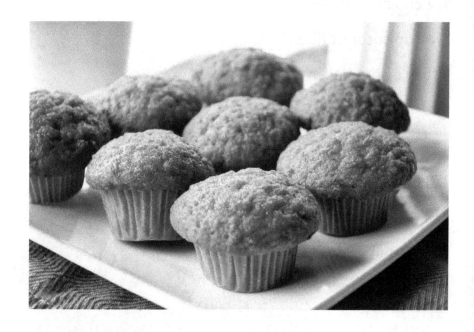

Preparation time: 15 minutes

Cooking time: 0 minutes

Servings: 6

Ingredients:

1 tsp cinnamon

2 tbsp coconut flour

20 drops liquid stevia

1/4 cup water

1/4 tsp vanilla extract

1/4 tsp baking soda

1/2 tsp baking powder

1/4 cup almond flour

1/2 cup ground flax

2 tbsp ground chia

Directions:

Warm oven to 350 F. Spray a muffin tray with cooking spray and set aside. Put 6 tablespoons of water and ground chia in a small bowl. Mix well and set aside.

In a mixing bowl, add ground flax, baking soda, baking powder, cinnamon, coconut flour, and almond flour and mix well.

Add chia seed mixture, vanilla, water, and liquid stevia and stir well to combine. Pour mixture into the prepared muffin tray and bake in preheated oven for 35 minutes. Serve and enjoy.

Nutrition:Calories 92, Fat 6.3 g, Carbohydrates 6.9 g, Protein 3.7 g

Grain-Free Overnight Oats

Preparation time: 15 minutes

Cooking time: 0 minutes

Servings: 1

Ingredients:

2/3 cup unsweetened coconut milk

2 tsp chia seeds

2 tbsp vanilla protein powder

½ tbsp coconut flour

3 tbsp hemp hearts

Directions:

Add all ingredients into the glass jar and stir to combine. Close jar with lid and place in the refrigerator overnight. Top with fresh berries and serve.

Nutrition:

Calories 378

Fat 22.5 g

Carbohydrates 15 g

Protein 27 g

Lunch Recipes

Tahini Broccoli

Preparation Time: 5 Minutes

Cooking Time: 15 Minutes

Servings: 4

Ingredients:

Toasted sesame seeds (.25 c.)

Minced green onions

Broccoli slaw (1 bag)

Soy sauce (2 teaspoon.)

Sesame oil (1 Tablespoon.)

Rice vinegar (1 Tablespoon.)

White miso (2 Tablespoon.)

Tahini (.25 c.)

Directions:

Take out a bowl and whisk together the soy sauce, oil, vinegar, miso, and tahini.

Add in the sesame seeds, green onions, and broccoli slaw. Set aside for 20 minutes and then serve.

Nutrition: Calories: 135 Carbs: 37g Fat: 0g Protein: 23g

Cauliflower Tacos

Preparation Time: 10 Minutes

Cooking Time: 30 Minutes

Servings: 8

Ingredients:

For the roasted cauliflower

Chili powder (1 teaspoon.)

Smoked paprika (2 teaspoon.)

Nutritional yeast (2 Tablespoon.)

Flour (2 Tablespoon.)

Olive oil (1 Tablespoon.)

Cauliflower (1 head)

For the tacos

Lime wedges (

Corn tortillas (8)

Guacamole (.5 c.)

Mango salsa (.5 c.)

Grated carrots (

Quartered cherry tomatoes (2 c.)

Shredded lettuce (2 c.)

Directions:

Turn on the oven and let it heat up to 350 degrees. Prepare a baking tray and set it to the side.

Toss the cauliflower with the oil and, in another bowl, mix all of the seasonings before adding it to the cauliflower.

Spread this onto the baking tray and add to the oven. After 20 minutes, this will be done, and you can take it out of the oven.

When the cauliflower is cooked, you can use those and the rest of the Ingredients: to assemble the tacos.

Nutrition: Calories: 198 Carbs: 32g Fat: 6g Protein: 7g

Sweet Potatoes

Preparation Time: 10 Minutes

Cooking Time: 35 Minutes

Servings: 4

Ingredients:

Salt (.5 teaspoon.)

Garlic powder (.5 teaspoon.)

Dried thyme (.5 teaspoon.)

Dried oregano (.5 teaspoon.)

Smoked paprika (.5 teaspoon.)

Cayenne pepper (.5 teaspoon.)

Olive oil (2 teaspoon.)

Sweet potatoes (2 lbs.)

Directions:

Turn on the oven and let it heat up to 400 degrees. Prepare a baking sheet with some parchment paper.

Wash the potatoes and then cube up. Move to a bowl and add the oil and potatoes together.

Combine the seasonings into another bowl and then sprinkle on top of the potatoes. Add this to the baking sheet and into the oven.

After 30 minutes of baking, take out of the oven and then serve warm.

Nutrition: Calories: 219 Carbs: 46g Fat: 3g Protein: 4g

Smoky Meal

Preparation Time: 5 Minutes

Cooking Time: 10 Minutes

Servings: 6

Ingredients:

Chipotle powder (.25 teaspoon.)

Smoked paprika (.25 teaspoon.)

Pepper (.25 teaspoon.)

Salt (.5 teaspoon.)

Plain vegan yogurt (3 Tablespoon.)

Rice vinegar (.25 c.)

Mayo (.33 c.)

Shredded cabbage (1 lb.)

Directions:

Bring out a big bowl and add the shredded cabbage inside. In another bowl, combine the chipotle powder, paprika, pepper, salt, sugar, yogurt, vinegar, and mayo.

Pour this over the cabbage and then mix it all up. Divide up and serve.

Nutrition: Calories: 73 Carbs: 8g Protein: 1g Fat: 4g

Dinner Recipes

Dijon Maple Burgers

Preparation Time: 20 minutes

Cooking Time: 30 minutes

Servings: 12

Ingredients:

1 Red Bell Pepper

19 ounces Can Chickpeas, rinsed & drained

1 cup Almonds, ground

2 teaspoons Dijon Mustard

1 teaspoon Oregano

½ teaspoon Sage

1 cup Spinach, fresh

1 – ½ cups Rolled Oats

1 Clove Garlic, pressed

½ Lemon, juiced

2 teaspoons Maple Syrup, pure

Directions:

Get out a baking sheet. Line it with parchment paper.

Cut your red pepper in half and then take the seeds out. Place it on your baking sheet, and roast in the oven while you prepare your other ingredients.

Process your chickpeas, almonds, mustard, and maple syrup together in a food processor.

Add in your lemon juice, oregano, sage, garlic, and spinach, processing again. Make sure it's combined, but don't puree it.

Once your red bell pepper is softened, which should roughly take ten minutes, add this to the processor as well. Add in your oats, mixing well.

Form twelve patties, cooking in the oven for a half-hour. They should be browned.

Nutrition:

Calories: 96 kcal

Protein: 5.28 g

Fat: 2.42 g

Carbohydrates: 16.82 g

Hearty Black Lentil Curry

Preparation Time: 30 minutes

Cooking Time: 6 hours and 15 minutes

Servings: 4

Ingredients:

1 cup of black lentils, rinsed and soaked overnight

14 ounces of chopped tomatoes

2 large white onions, peeled and sliced

1 1/2 teaspoon of minced garlic

1 teaspoon of grated ginger

1 red chili

1 teaspoon of salt

1/4 teaspoon of red chili powder

1 teaspoon of paprika

1 teaspoon of ground turmeric

2 teaspoons of ground cumin

2 teaspoons of ground coriander

1/2 cup of chopped coriander

4-ounce of vegetarian butter

4 fluid of ounce water

2 fluid of ounce vegetarian double cream

Directions:

Place a large pan over moderate heat, add butter and let heat until melt.

Add the onion and garlic and ginger and cook for 10 to 15 minutes or until onions are caramelized.

Then stir in salt, red chili powder, paprika, turmeric, cumin, ground coriander, and water.

Transfer this mixture to a 6-quarts slow cooker and add tomatoes and red chili.

Drain lentils, add to slow cooker, and stir until just mix.

Plugin slow cooker; adjust cooking time to 6 hours and let cook on low heat setting.

When the lentils are done, stir in cream and adjust the seasoning.

Serve with boiled rice or whole wheat bread.

Nutrition: Calories: 299 kcal , Protein: 5.59 g , Fat: 27.92 g , Carbohydrates: 9.83 g

Flavorful Refried Beans

Preparation Time: 15 minutes

Cooking Time: 8 hours

Servings: 8

Ingredients:

3 cups of pinto beans, rinsed

1 small jalapeno pepper, seeded and chopped

1 medium-sized white onion, peeled and sliced

2 tablespoons of minced garlic

5 teaspoons of salt

2 teaspoons of ground black pepper

1/4 teaspoon of ground cumin

9 cups of water

Directions:

Using a 6-quarts slow cooker, place all the ingredients and stir until it mixes properly.

Cover the top, plug in the slow cooker, adjust the cooking time to 6 hours, let it cook on the high heat setting, and add more water if the beans get too dry.

When the beans are done, drain it then reserve the liquid.

Mash the beans using a potato masher and pour in the reserved cooking liquid until it reaches your desired mixture.

Serve immediately.

Nutrition:

Calories: 268 kcal

Protein: 16.55 g

Fat: 1.7 g

Carbohydrates: 46.68 g

Smoky Red Beans and Rice

Preparation Time: 15 minutes

Cooking Time: 6 minutes

Servings: 6

Ingredients:

30 ounces of cooked red beans

1 cup of brown rice, uncooked

1 cup of chopped green pepper

1 cup of chopped celery

1 cup of chopped white onion

1 1/2 teaspoon of minced garlic

1/2 teaspoon of salt

1/4 teaspoon of cayenne pepper

1 teaspoon of smoked paprika

2 teaspoons of dried thyme

1 bay leaf

2 1/3 cups of vegetable broth

Directions:

Using a 6-quarts slow cooker, place all the ingredients except for the rice, salt, and cayenne pepper.

Stir until it mixes properly and then cover the top.

Plug in the slow cooker, adjust the cooking time to 4 hours, and steam on a low heat setting.

Then pour in and stir the rice, salt, cayenne pepper and continue cooking for an additional 2 hours at a high heat setting.

Serve straight away.

Nutrition:

Calories: 791 kcal

Protein: 3.25 g

Fat: 86.45 g

Carbohydrates: 9.67 g

Vegetables Recipes

Steamed Cauliflower

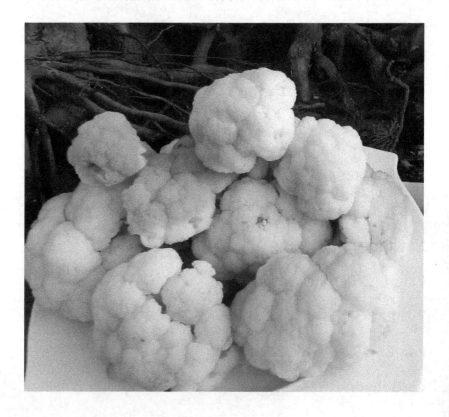

Preparation Time: 5 minutes

Cooking Time: 10 minutes

Servings: 6

Ingredients:

1 large head cauliflower

1 cup water

½ teaspoon salt

1 teaspoon red pepper flakes (optional)

Directions:

Remove any leaves from the cauliflower, and cut it into florets.

In a large saucepan, bring the water to a boil. Place a steamer basket over the water, and add the florets and salt. Cover and steam for 5 to 7 minutes, until tender. In a large bowl, toss the cauliflower with the red pepper flakes (if using). Transfer the florets to a large airtight container or 6 single-serving containers. Let cool before sealing the lids.

Nutrition:

Calories: 35; Fat: 0g; Protein: 3g; Carbohydrates: 7g; Fiber: 4g; Sugar: 4g; Sodium: 236mg

Cajun Sweet Potatoes

Preparation Time: 5 minutes

Cooking Time: 30 minutes

Servings: 4

Ingredients:

2 pounds' sweet potatoes

2 teaspoons extra-virgin olive oil

½ teaspoon ground cayenne pepper

½ teaspoon smoked paprika

½ teaspoon dried oregano

½ teaspoon dried thyme

½ teaspoon garlic powder

½ teaspoon salt (optional)

Directions:

Preheat the oven to 400ºF. Line a baking sheet with parchment paper.

Wash the potatoes, pat dry, and cut into ¾-inch cubes. Transfer to a large bowl, and pour the olive oil over the potatoes.

In a small bowl, combine the cayenne, paprika, oregano, thyme, and garlic powder. Sprinkle the spices over the potatoes and combine until the potatoes are well coated. Spread the potatoes on the prepared baking sheet in a single layer. Season with the salt (if using). Roast for 30 minutes, stirring the potatoes after 15 minutes.

Divide the potatoes evenly among 4 single-serving containers. Let cool completely before sealing.

Nutrition:

Calories: 219; Fat: 3g; Protein: 4g; Carbohydrates: 46g; Fiber: 7g; Sugar: 9g; Sodium: 125mg

Smoky Coleslaw

Preparation Time: 10 minutes

Cooking Time: 0 minute

Servings: 6

Ingredients:

1-pound shredded cabbage

1/3 cup vegan mayonnaise

¼ cup unseasoned rice vinegar

3 tablespoons plain vegan yogurt or plain soymilk

1 tablespoon vegan sugar

½ teaspoon salt

¼ teaspoon freshly ground black pepper

¼ teaspoon smoked paprika

¼ teaspoon chipotle powder

Directions:

Put the shredded cabbage in a large bowl. In a medium bowl, whisk the mayonnaise, vinegar, yogurt, sugar, salt, pepper, paprika, and chipotle powder.

Pour over the cabbage, and mix with a spoon or spatula until the cabbage shreds are coated. Divide the coleslaw evenly among 6 single-serving containers. Seal the lids.

Nutrition:

Calories: 73; Fat: 4g; Protein: 1g; Carbohydrates: 8g; Fiber: 2g; Sugar: 5g; Sodium: 283mg

Mediterranean Hummus Pizza

Preparation Time: 10 minutes

Cooking Time: 30 minutes

Servings: 2 pizzas

Ingredients:

½ zucchini, thinly sliced

½ red onion, thinly sliced

1 cup cherry tomatoes, halved

2 to 4 tablespoons pitted and chopped black olives

Pinch sea salt

Drizzle olive oil (optional)

2 prebaked pizza crusts

½ cup Classic Hummus

2 to 4 tablespoons Cheesy Sprinkle

Directions:

Preheat the oven to 400°F. Place the zucchini, onion, cherry tomatoes, and olives in a large bowl, sprinkle them with the sea salt, and toss them a bit. Drizzle with a bit of olive oil (if using), seal in the flavor and keep them from drying out in the oven.

Lay the two crusts out on a large baking sheet. Spread half the hummus on each crust, and top with the veggie mixture and some Cheesy Sprinkle. Pop the pizzas in the oven for 20 to 30 minutes, or until the veggies are soft.

Nutrition:

Calories: 500; Total fat: 25g; Carbs: 58g; Fiber: 12g; Protein:

Finger Food

Balls from Beetroot

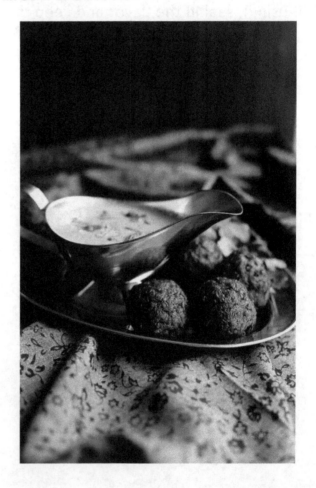

Preparation time: 35 minutes

Cooking time: 0 minutes

Servings: 4

Ingredients:

4 sprigs of parsley

2 tablespoon walnuts

260 g beetroot

½ onion

1 clove of garlic

Salt and pepper

Directions:

Boil the beetroot, peel and grate coarsely with a kitchen grater.

Roast the walnuts and process them into flour in a food processor.

Cut the onion into small cubes, peel the garlic clove and mash it with a fork.

Wash, shake and chop the parsley.

Mix all Ingredients: in a bowl and season with salt and a little pepper.

Shape into balls of the same size and let stand for a few minutes.

Nutrition:

Calories: 239

Fat: 11.4g

Carbs: 10.5g

Protein: 12.1g

Fiber: 3.2g

Polenta Skewers

Preparation time: 35 minutes

Cooking time: 0 minutes

Servings: 4

Ingredients:

½ avocado

10 cherry tomatoes

1 mini zucchini

150 g corn grits

2 tablespoon olive oil

1 teaspoon sesame seeds, black

10 basil leaves

10 toothpicks

450 ml vegetable stock

Salt and pepper

Directions:

The day before, bring the corn grits to the boil in the broth and cook for a few minutes, stirring constantly. Pour into a square form and chill until the next day.

Cut the polenta into small cubes and fry in a pan in a little olive oil.

Wash the zucchini, cut into thin slices and fry in the pan once the polenta is ready.

Wash the tomatoes and cut them in half, pluck the basil leaves from the branches.

Stone the avocado and cut into thin slices.

Skewer a polenta cube, a zucchini, a tomato, a slice of avocado and a basil leaf onto a toothpick. Serve with sesame seeds.

Nutrition:

Calories: 259

Fat: 15.4g

Carbs: 20.5g

Protein: 12.1g

Fiber: 3.2g

Börek with Spinach Filling

Preparation time: 25 minutes

Cooking time: 0 minutes

Servings: 10

Ingredients:

10 yufka sheets

2 cloves of garlic

1 small onion

3 tablespoon soy yogurts

4 tablespoon soy milk

400 g spinach

3 tablespoons of oil

1 pinch of nutmeg

Salt and pepper

Directions:

Wash the spinach, peel the garlic and onion and cut into small cubes.

Steam the spinach, onion and garlic in oil in a deep pan.

After a few minutes, season with nutmeg, salt and pepper and stir in the yoghurt.

Lay out the Yufka leaves and brush with the spinach filling.

Roll up and brush with a little milk.

Then place on a baking sheet and bake in the oven at 180 degrees Celsius for about 15 minutes.

Nutrition:

Calories: 219

Fat: 9.4g

Carbs: 10.5g

Protein: 11.1g

Fiber: 3.2g

Taler With Avocado Cream

Preparation time: 25 minutes

Cooking time: 0 minutes

Servings: 5

Ingredients:

20 pumpernickels, round

1 chili pepper

1 lime

2 avocados

6 beetroot chips

50 g vegan cream cheese

Salt and pepper

Directions:

Cut the chili pepper lengthways and scrape out the stones.

Halve the avocados, core them and scrape the pulp into a blender jar.

Add the cream cheese and a little lime juice.

Mix a homogeneous cream from the chili pepper, avocado, lime, cream cheese and a little salt and pepper.

Put the little Pumpernickel Taler ready and put a serving of avocado cream on each with a piping bag.

Crumble the chips and sprinkle them over the thalers.

Nutrition:

Calories: 243

Fat: 10.4g

Carbs: 12.5g

Protein: 9.1g

Fiber: 3.2g

Small Sweet Potato Pancakes

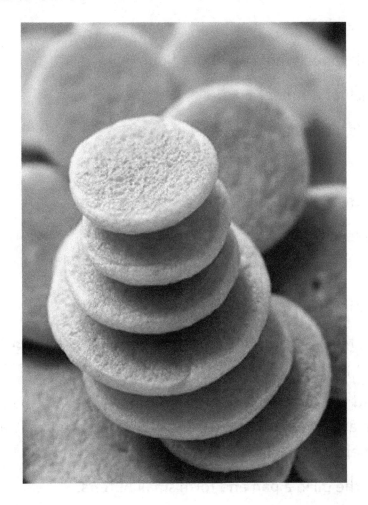

Preparation time: 20 minutes

Cooking time: 0 minutes

Servings: 2

Ingredients:

1 clove of garlic

3 tablespoon whole meal rice flour

1 pinch of nutmeg

3 tablespoons of water

150 g sweet potato

1 pinch of chili flakes

1 teaspoon oil

Salt

Directions:

Peel the garlic clove and mash it with a fork. Peel the sweet potato and grate it into small sticks with a grater.

Knead the sweet potato and garlic in a bowl with the rice flour and water, then season with chili flakes, salt and nutmeg.

Heat the oil in a pan and form small buffers.

Fry these in the pan on both sides until golden brown.

Goes perfectly with tzatziki and other fresh dips.

Nutrition: Calories: 209 Fat: 15.4g Carbs: 10.5g Protein: 8.1g Fiber: 3.2g

Pumpernickel with Avocado

Preparation time: 10 minutes

Cooking time: 0 minutes

Servings: 2

Ingredients:

6 small slices of pumpernickel

1 avocado

1 roll of vegan cheese spread

1 tablespoon chives

Salt and pepper

Directions:

Halve the avocado, remove the seeds and carefully remove from the skin. Cut into slices and place on a plate.

Spread cheese on the bread, then top with avocado and then sprinkle with a little pepper and chopped chives.

Nutrition:

Calories: 159

Fat: 9.4g

Carbs: 10.5g

Protein: 9.1g

Fiber: 3.2g

Mushroom Cakes

Preparation time: 30 minutes

Cooking time: 0 minutes

Servings: 4

Ingredients:

1 bun

1 small onion

1 clove of garlic

500 g mushrooms

1 pinch of marjoram

2 tablespoons of oil

1 tablespoon flaxseed, crushed

3 tablespoon soy milk

Salt and pepper

Directions:

Clean the mushrooms and cut into small cubes. Peel the onion and garlic, then also dice.

Crumble the bun and mix in a bowl with the mushrooms, garlic and onion.

Add marjoram, salt and pepper and fold in the flax seeds as well.

Add soy milk so that the mixture sticks well.

Heat the oil in a non-stick pan, form small meatballs and fry them until golden brown on both sides.

Nutrition:

Calories: 129

Fat: 12.4g

Carbs: 11.5g

Protein: 9.1g

Fiber: 3.2g

Churros with Chocolate

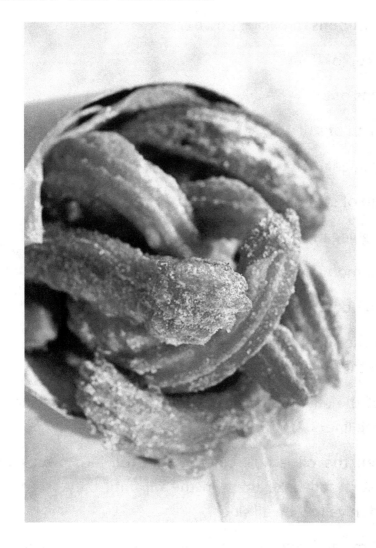

Preparation time: 35 minutes

Cooking time: 0 minutes

Servings: 6

Ingredients:

2 teaspoons of baking powder

1 ¼ cup of flour

2 cups of oil

1 pinch of salt

50 g sugar

1 cup of soy milk

100 g vegan chocolate

cinnamon and sugar

Directions:

Mix the sugar, baking powder, flour and salt. Then stir in ¾ of the soy milk until a velvety batter is formed.

Heat the oil in a saucepan and roll the churro batter into a long line.

When the oil is hot, cut the thin roll into pieces with scissors and bake them in the oil until they are evenly golden yellow on all sides.

In Zimt and roll sugar and heat the chocolate with the remaining soy milk.

Nutrition: Calories: 209 Fat: 15.4g Carbs: 20.5g Protein: 12.1g Fiber: 3.2g

Zucchini Rolls with Cream Cheese

Preparation time: 35 minutes

Cooking time: 0 minutes

Servings: 4

Ingredients:

1 tablespoon oil

60 g apricots, dried

350 g zucchini

Salt and pepper

1 sprig of thyme

½ lime

Directions:

Turn after a minute and fry the same way on the other side.

Let cool on a plate and in the meantime prepare the filling.

Let the apricots soak a little and then chop them.

Mix with the cream cheese, chopped thyme and a little pepper. Season to taste with salt and prepare.

Brush the zucchini slices with some filling and roll up.

Add a few squirts of lime juice to serve.

Nutrition: Calories: 235 Fat: 15.4g Carbs: 20.5g Protein: 12.1g Fiber: 3.2g

Soup and Stew

Cabbage & Beet Stew

Preparation Time: 20 minutes

Cooking Time: 10 minutes

Servings: 4

Ingredients:

2 Tablespoons Olive Oil

3 Cups Vegetable Broth

2 Tablespoons Lemon Juice, Fresh

½ Teaspoon Garlic Powder

½ Cup Carrots, Shredded

2 Cups Cabbage, Shredded

1 Cup Beets, Shredded

Dill for Garnish

½ Teaspoon Onion Powder

Sea Salt & Black Pepper to Taste

Directions:

Heat oil in a pot, and then sauté your vegetables.

Pour your broth in, mixing in your seasoning. Simmer until it's cooked through, and then top with dill.

Nutrition:

kcal: 263

Carbohydrates: 8 g

Protein: 20.3 g

Fat: 24 g

Basil Tomato Soup

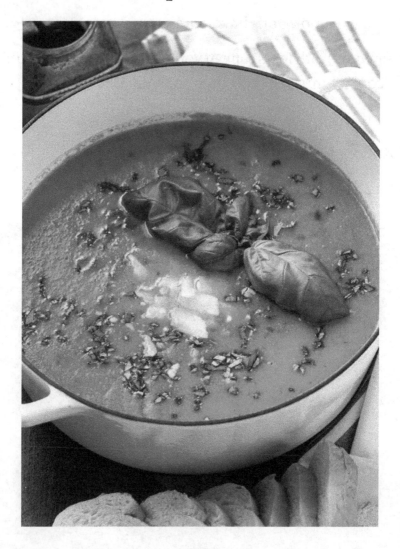

Preparation Time: 10 minutes

Cooking Time: 10 minutes

Servings: 6

Ingredients:

28 oz can tomato

¼ cup basil pesto

¼ tsp dried basil leaves

1 tsp apple cider vinegar

2 tbsp erythritol

¼ tsp garlic powder

½ tsp onion powder

2 cups water

1 ½ tsp kosher salt

Directions:

Add tomatoes, garlic powder, onion powder, water, and salt in a saucepan.

Bring to boil over medium heat. Reduce heat and simmer for 2 minutes.

Remove saucepan from heat and puree the soup using a blender until smooth.

Stir in pesto, dried basil, vinegar, and erythritol.

Stir well and serve warm.

Nutrition: kcal: 662 Carbohydrates: 18 g Protein: 8 g Fat: 55 g

Mushroom & Broccoli Soup

Preparation Time: 20 minutes

Cooking Time: 45 minutes

Servings: 8

Ingredients:

1 bundle broccoli (around 1-1/2 pounds)

1 tablespoon canola oil

1/2 pound cut crisp mushrooms

1 tablespoon diminished sodium soy sauce

2 medium carrots, finely slashed

2 celery ribs, finely slashed

1/4 cup finely slashed onion

1 garlic clove, minced

1 container (32 ounces) vegetable juices

2 cups of water

2 tablespoons lemon juice

Directions:

Cut broccoli florets into reduced down pieces. Strip and hack stalks.

In an enormous pot, heat oil over medium-high warmth; sauté mushrooms until delicate, 4-6 minutes. Mix in soy sauce; expel from skillet.

In the same container, join broccoli stalks, carrots, celery, onion, garlic, soup, and water; heat to the point of boiling. Diminish heat; stew, revealed, until vegetables are relaxed, 25-30 minutes.

Puree soup utilizing a drenching blender. Or then again, cool marginally, puree the soup in a blender; come back to the dish.

Mix in florets and mushrooms; heat to the point of boiling. Lessen warmth to medium; cook until broccoli is delicate, 8-10 minutes, blending infrequently. Mix in lemon juice.

Nutrition:

kcal: 830

Carbohydrates: 8 g

Protein: 45 g

Fat: 64 g

Appetizer

Nacho Kale Chips

Preparation time: 10 minutes

Cooking time: 14 hours

Servings: 10

Ingredients:

2 bunches of curly kale

2 cups cashews, soaked, drained

1/2 cup chopped red bell pepper

1 teaspoon garlic powder

1 teaspoon salt

2 tablespoons red chili powder

1/2 teaspoon smoked paprika

1/2 cup nutritional yeast

1 teaspoon cayenne

3 tablespoons lemon juice

3/4 cup water

Directions:

Place all the ingredients except for kale in a food processor and pulse for 2 minutes until smooth.

Place kale in a large bowl, pour in the blended mixture, mix until coated, and dehydrate for 14 hours at 120 degrees F until crispy.

If dehydrator is not available, spread kale between two baking sheets and bake for 90 minutes at 225 degrees F until crispy, flipping halfway. When done, let chips cool for 15 minutes and then serve.

Nutrition:

Calories: 191

Fat: 12 g

Carbs: 16 g

Protein: 9 g

Red Salsa

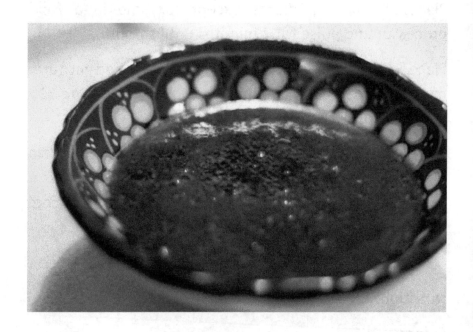

Preparation time: 10 minutes

Cooking time: 0 minute

Servings: 8

Ingredients:

30 ounces diced fire-roasted tomatoes

4 tablespoons diced green chilies

1 medium jalapeño pepper, deseeded

1/2 cup chopped green onion

1 cup chopped cilantro

1 teaspoon minced garlic

½ teaspoon of sea salt

1 teaspoon ground cumin

¼ teaspoon stevia

3 tablespoons lime juice

Directions:

Place all the fixings in a food processor and process for 2 minutes until smooth. Tip the salsa in a bowl, taste to adjust seasoning and then serve.

Nutrition:

Calories: 71

Fat: 0.2 g

Carbs: 19 g

Protein: 2 g

Tomato Hummus

Preparation time: 5 minutes

Cooking time: 0 minute

Servings: 4

Ingredients:

1/4 cup sun-dried tomatoes, without oil

1 ½ cups cooked chickpeas

1 teaspoon minced garlic

1/2 teaspoon salt

2 tablespoons sesame oil

1 tablespoon lemon juice

1 tablespoon olive oil

1/4 cup of water

Directions:

Place all the fixings in a food processor and process for 2 minutes until smooth.

Tip the hummus in a bowl, drizzle with more oil, and then serve straight away.

Nutrition:Calories: 122.7 Fat: 4.1 g Carbs: 17.8 g Protein: 5.1 g

Marinated Mushrooms

Preparation time: 10 minutes

Cooking time: 7 minutes

Servings: 6

Ingredients:

12 ounces small button mushrooms

1 teaspoon minced garlic

1/4 teaspoon dried thyme

1/2 teaspoon sea salt

1/2 teaspoon dried basil

1/2 teaspoon red pepper flakes

1/4 teaspoon dried oregano

1/2 teaspoon maple syrup

1/4 cup apple cider vinegar

1/4 cup and 1 teaspoon olive oil

2 tablespoons chopped parsley

Directions:

Take a skillet pan, place it over medium-high heat, add 1 teaspoon oil and when hot, add mushrooms and cook for 5 minutes until golden brown.

Meanwhile, prepare the marinade and for this, place remaining ingredients in a bowl and whisk until combined.

When mushrooms have cooked, transfer them into the bowl of marinade and toss until well coated. Serve straight away

Nutrition:

Calories: 103

Fat: 9 g

Carbs: 2 g

Protein: 1 g

Drinks

Banana Weight Loss Juice

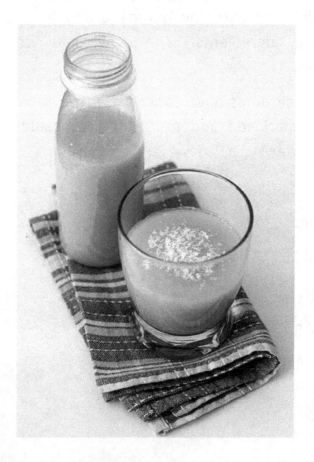

Preparation Time: 10 Minutes

Cooking Time: 0 Minutes

Servings: 1

Ingredients:

Water (1/3 C.)

Apple (1, Sliced)

Orange (1, Sliced)

Banana (1, Sliced)

Lemon Juice (1 T.)

Directions:

Looking to boost your weight loss? The key is taking in less calories; this recipe can get you there.

Simply place everything into your blender, blend on high for twenty seconds, and then pour into your glass.

Nutrition: Calories: 289 Total Carbohydrate: 2 g Cholesterol: 3 mg Total Fat: 17 g Fiber: 2 g Protein: 7 g Sodium: 163 mg

Citrus Detox Juice

Preparation Time: 10 Minutes

Cooking Time: 0 Minutes

Servings: 4

Ingredients:

Water (3 C.)

Lemon (1, Sliced)

Grapefruit (1, Sliced)

Orange (1, Sliced)

Directions:

While starting your new diet, it is going to be vital to stay hydrated. This detox juice is the perfect solution and offers some extra flavor.

Begin by peeling and slicing up your fruit. Once this is done, place in a pitcher of water and infuse the water overnight.

Nutrition: Calories: 269 Total Carbohydrate: 2 g Cholesterol: 3 mg Total Fat: 14 g Fiber: 2 g Protein: 7 g Sodium: 183 mg

Metabolism Water

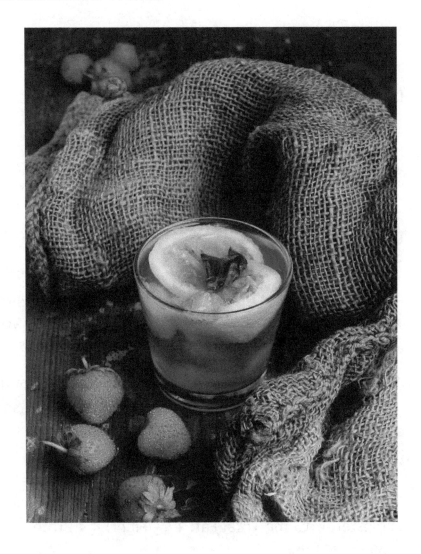

Preparation Time: 10 Minutes

Cooking Time: 0 Minutes

Servings: 1

Ingredients:

Water (3 C.)

Cucumber (1, Sliced)

Lemon (1, Sliced)

Mint (2 Leaves)

Ice

Directions:

At some point, we probably all wish for a quicker metabolism! With the lemon acting as an energizer, cucumber for a refreshing taste, and mint to help your stomach digest, this water is perfect!

All you will have to do is get out a pitcher, place all of the ingredients in, and allow the ingredients to soak overnight for maximum benefits!

Nutrition: Calories: 301 Total Carbohydrate: 2 g Cholesterol: 13 mg Total Fat: 17 g Fiber: 4 g Protein: 8 g Sodium: 201 mg

Stress Relief Detox Drink

Preparation Time: 5 Minutes

Cooking Time: 0 Minutes

Servings: 1

Ingredients:

Water (1 Pitcher)

Mint   1

Lemon (1, Sliced)

Basil 1

Strawberries (1 C., Sliced)

Ice 2

Directions:

Life can be a pretty stressful event. Luckily, there is water to help keep you cool, calm, and collected! The lemon works like an energizer, the basil is a natural antidepressant, and mint can help your stomach do its job better. As for the strawberries, those are just for some sweetness!

When you are ready, take all of the ingredients and place into a pitcher of water overnight and enjoy the next day.

Nutrition: Calories: 189 Total Carbohydrate: 2 g Cholesterol: 73 mg Total Fat: 17 g Fiber: 0 g Protein: 7 g Sodium: 163 mg

Dessert Recipes

Apple Crumble

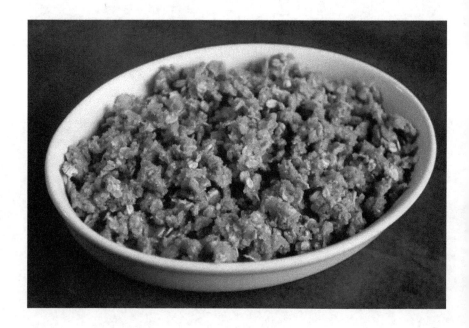

Preparation Time: 20 minutes

Cooking Time: 25 minutes

Servings: 6

Ingredients:

For the filling

4 to 5 apples, cored and chopped (about 6 cups)

½ cup unsweetened applesauce, or ¼ cup water

2 to 3 tablespoons unrefined sugar (coconut, date, sucanat, maple syrup)

1 teaspoon ground cinnamon

Pinch sea salt

For the crumble

2 tablespoons almond butter, or cashew or sunflower seed butter

2 tablespoons maple syrup

1½ cups rolled oats

½ cup walnuts, finely chopped

½ teaspoon ground cinnamon

2 to 3 tablespoons unrefined granular sugar (coconut, date, sucanat)

Directions:

Preparing the Ingredients.

Preheat the oven to 350°F. Put the apples and applesauce in an 8-inch-square baking dish, and sprinkle with the sugar, cinnamon, and salt. Toss to combine.

In a medium bowl, mix the nut butter and maple syrup until smooth and creamy. Add the oats, walnuts, cinnamon, and sugar and stir to coat, using your hands if necessary. (If you have a small food processor, pulse the oats and walnuts together before adding them to the mix.)

Sprinkle the topping over the apples, and put the dish in the oven.

Bake for 20 to 25 minutes, or until the fruit is soft and the topping is lightly browned.

Nutrition: Calories 195 Fat 7 g Carbohydrates 6 g Sugar 2 g Protein 24 g Cholesterol 65 mg

Cashew-Chocolate Truffles

Preparation Time: 15 minutes

Cooking Time: 0 minutes

Servings: 12

Ingredients:

1 cup raw cashews, soaked in water overnight

¾ cup pitted dates

2 tablespoons coconut oil

1 cup unsweetened shredded coconut, divided

1 to 2 tablespoons cocoa powder, to taste

Directions:

Preparing the Ingredients.

In a food processor, combine the cashews, dates, coconut oil, ½ cup of shredded coconut, and cocoa powder. Pulse until fully incorporated; it will resemble chunky cookie dough. Spread the remaining ½ cup of shredded coconut on a plate.

Form the mixture into tablespoon-size balls and roll on the plate to cover with the shredded coconut. Transfer to a parchment paper–lined plate or baking sheet. Repeat to make 12 truffles.

Place the truffles in the refrigerator for 1 hour to set. Transfer the truffles to a storage container or freezer-safe bag and seal.

Nutrition: Calories 160 Fat 1 g Carbohydrates 1 g Sugar 0.5 g Protein 22 g Cholesterol 60 mg

Banana Chocolate Cupcakes

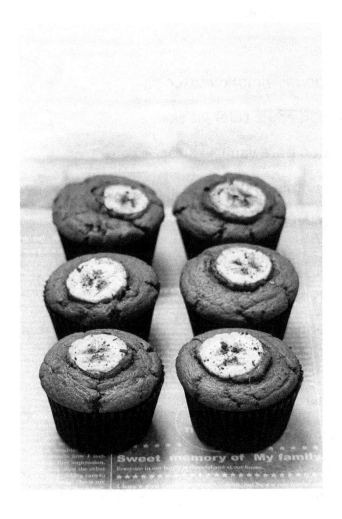

Preparation Time: 20 minutes

Cooking Time: 20 minutes

Servings: 1

Ingredients:

3 medium bananas

1 cup non-dairy milk

2 tablespoons almond butter

1 teaspoon apple cider vinegar

1 teaspoon pure vanilla extract

1¼ cups whole-grain flour

½ cup rolled oats

¼ cup coconut sugar (optional)

1 teaspoon baking powder

½ teaspoon baking soda

½ cup unsweetened cocoa powder

¼ cup chia seeds, or sesame seeds

Pinch sea salt

¼ cup dark chocolate chips, dried cranberries, or raisins (optional)

Directions:

Preparing the Ingredients.

Preheat the oven to 350°F. Lightly grease the cups of two 6-cup muffin tins or line with paper muffin cups.

Put the bananas, milk, almond butter, vinegar, and vanilla in a blender and purée until smooth. Or stir together in a large bowl until smooth and creamy.

Put the flour, oats, sugar (if using), baking powder, baking soda, cocoa powder, chia seeds, salt, and chocolate chips in another large bowl, and stir to combine. Mix the wet and dry ingredients, stirring as little as possible. Spoon into muffin cups, and bake for 20 to 25 minutes. Take the cupcakes out of the oven and let them cool fully before taking out of the muffin tins, since they'll be very moist.

Nutrition: Calories 295 Fat 17 g Carbohydrates 4 g Sugar 0.1 g Protein 29 g Cholesterol 260 mg

Minty Fruit Salad

Preparation Time: 15 minutes

Cooking Time: 5 minutes

Servings: 4

Ingredients:

¼ cup lemon juice (about 2 small lemons)

4 teaspoons maple syrup or agave syrup

2 cups chopped pineapple

2 cups chopped strawberries

2 cups raspberries

1 cup blueberries

8 fresh mint leaves

Directions:

Preparing the Ingredients.

Beginning with 1 mason jar, add the ingredients in this order:

1 tablespoon of lemon juice, 1 teaspoon of maple syrup, ½ cup of pineapple, ½ cup of strawberries, ½ cup of raspberries, ¼ cup of blueberries, and 2 mint leaves.

Repeat to fill 3 more jars. Close the jars tightly with lids.

Place the airtight jars in the refrigerator for up to 3 days.

Nutrition: Calories 339 Fat 17.5 g Carbohydrates 2 g Sugar 2 g Protein 44 g Cholesterol 100 mg

Conclusion

Congratulations on making it to the end of this cookbook. Eating more plant nutrients correlates with lifespan and decreased risk for most ongoing infections, including coronary heart disease and type 2 diabetes. Plant nutrients (e.g., whole grains, beans, organics, vegetables , nuts and seeds) are abundant for wellness that promotes supplements and blends such as nutrients, minerals, fiber and phytochemicals. Plants can also be a decent source of protein and I hope I have made this clear to you with my collection of recipes.

Now the next step is to learn how to change your lifestyle and your eating habits, to do so you just need to follow these recipes again and again.

Good luck!

9 781802 523669